Stop

Bedwetting

in 7 days

*A simple step-by-step guide to help
children conquer bedwetting problems
in just a few days*

ALICIA EATON

First edition published in 2009

© Copyright 2009

Alicia Eaton

Paperback ISBN 9781904312703

Published in the UK by MX Publishing

335 Princess Park Manor, Royal Drive,

London, N11 3GX

www.mxpublishing.co.uk

Cover Design by Staunch Design

www.staunch.com

Illustrations by Imogen McGuinness

"Alicia Eaton has a real gift for communicating complex ideas in a way that makes them easy to incorporate into your daily routine. I highly recommend her work, particularly when applied to children (and their parents!)"

Michael Neil bestselling author of 'You Can Have What You Want' and ''Supercoach'

"What a wonderful, practical, easy-to-read book. Alicia's common-sense approach, skills and experience – plus a liberal sprinkling of NLP techniques makes this a must-read book for parents.

Dr Stephen Simpson MB CHB MFOM MBA Medical Doctor and NLP Trainer

'Thank you for putting an end to my teenage daughter's misery....''

Vanessa Gottlieb, Parent

ABOUT THE AUTHOR

Alicia Eaton is a Clinical Hypnotherapist and Advanced Practitioner of NLP, trained by Richard Bandler (co-creator of NLP) and Paul McKenna.

She has been part of Paul McKenna's seminar assisting team for many years and has fine-tuned her coaching skills with Michael Neill, the renowned success coach.

As well as working with adults, she is now a recognised expert on the use of NLP and hypnosis with children and runs successful practices in both London and Hertfordshire.

A qualified Montessori Teacher, she was Principal of her own school for five years and went on to study Developmental Psychology at The Anna Freud Centre and University College London.

She lives in Hertfordshire and has three children.

ACKNOWLEDGEMENTS

The ideas and techniques used in this book are based on the principles of NLP co-created by **Richard Bandler**. I'd like to thank him for giving me his approval to develop these ideas further and use them to help children.

A big thank you to **Paul McKenna** for his support and for giving me the opportunity to watch and learn so much from him over the years.

I'd also like to thank **Michael Neill** for showing me how 'success can be easy'. **Mark Hayley, Gabe Guerrero** and **Eric Robbie –** thank you for putting the polish on my NLP skills.

Thanks also to **Steve Emecz** of MX Publishing, **Bob Gibson** of Staunch and **Brian Hubbard**, Studio 86 Photography. And **Imogen McGuinness** - for her fabulous illustrations!

My children - **George, Tom** and **Clementine** – for simply being the best kids anyone could wish for.

Last and, by no means least – my partner **Neil–** for his expertise in turning ideas into reality and for keeping me sane. Thank you.

CONTENTS

INTRODUCTION

If you have a child that wets the bed, you might be feeling as if you are the only parent in the world whose child has this unwanted habit. It can be difficult to discuss the subject with family and friends, leaving you at a loss to understand why your child has failed to stop a habit that so many other children seem to get over with ease.

If this sounds familiar, then take comfort from knowing that more than 750,000 children in the UK accidentally wet their beds at night. Bedwetting occurs on most nights in 15% of five year olds and is still a problem for 3% of all 15 year olds. The numbers are just an estimate of course, because bedwetting is not a subject that parents are happy to discuss openly. In many cases, it isn't even a subject that is talked about within the family.

The truth is that millions of children from all over the world, wet their beds or have to rely on protective pants every single night. If your child is one of them, it's very likely that there are at least one or two more in their class at school with the same problem.

You are not on your own and the good news is bedwetting can be easily overcome.

For a number of years, I have been helping parents and their children to conquer this habit. I have seen the consequences of bedwetting - children suffer from a lack of confidence and low self-esteem, often failing to achieve their full-potential. Invitations to sleep overs with other children have to be refused, school trips and camps are met with fear and family holidays are not the relaxing times they are meant to be.

Let me put your mind at ease by reassuring you that bedwetting can be cured and the positive effects on your child will be amazing. Solving your child's bedwetting problem is much more than just achieving night-time dryness - it is about giving your child an increase in their level of self-confidence both at home and at school, which can lead to improved performance in the classrom and better interaction with their peers.

My reason for writing this book is that I believe that the process I have successfully developed over a number of years can be easily learned by parents.

In order to solve problems we often need to *stop* things happening. And the best way to do this is to *think* carefully about what you do want to happen and then *plan* how to be successful.

I've done the work for you and devised a plan that will enable you and your child to achieve that success. The effects on your child once they've got rid of the bedwetting habit will be life-changing. The effects on you as a parent will be equally liberating and rejuvenating!

My system incorporates the latest techniques and success strategies from the fields of hypnotherapy and NLP (Neuro-linguistic Programming). People are often surprised when I tell them that I regularly see children for hypnotherapy sessions. We're used to hearing about the use of hypnotherapy to help adults quit smoking or lose weight, but what's less known is that these same techniques can be used very safely and effectively with children.

These techniques complement a child's natural development and encourage those vital mind and body connections to be made. Once these are established, there's no looking back – you'll have dry nights forever.

I've been able to develop this system as a result of being trained by three of the world's experts in the field of 'success and changework'. Collectively, Richard Bandler (the co-creator of NLP), Paul McKenna and Michael Neill have enabled thousands of people to change their lives for the better.   I've worked alongside them for over 5 years and studied their methods in detail.

In this book, I'm going to show you how easy it is to apply these very same techniques and success strategies to this widespread and common childhood problem.   In just a week, you'll have mastered some of the techniques that will enable you to enjoy the life-changing benefits that achieving night-time dryness will have on you and your family.

Changes will be noticeable in days and the benefits will be felt for years.

And keep checking my website too because you'll find some extra Bedwetting tips here.

(www.aliciaeaton.co.uk)

CHAPTER ONE

•

Bedwetting – what's it all about?

BEDWETTING – WHAT'S IT ALL ABOUT?

Before we look at how hypnotherapy and NLP could help you and your child, let's have a look in more detail at what this problem is all about.

Bedwetting – also known as nocturnal enuresis – affects most children up to the age of three as the development of bladder function control can be a slow process. Bedwetting can continue to be quite common in children up the age of eight and sometimes even into their teenage years.

Studies show that bedwetting children who are given professional help and advice are more likely to become dry than those who aren't. With one or two children in every 100 failing to achieve night-time dryness, it is vitally important to get help at the right time. Some children never quite 'grow out' of their bedwetting habit, often carrying the scars into adulthood. Prolonged childhood bedwetting can manifest itself in many ways: difficulties forming relationships and getting jobs, susceptibility to stress, anxiety and even depression.

HOW COMMON IS BEDWETTING?

Bedwetting is a common problem, especially in the under-fives. According to figures published by the British Medical Journal, at the age of five as many as 20 children in 100 will have difficulty in controlling their bladders at night-time.

By age seven, this figure has dropped to around eight children in every 100, so we can see that most children will develop that vital mind/body link at around the age of six years.

It's at this age that children enter a new developmental phase. A good indicator of this happening is the loss of milk teeth. If your child still wets the bed at night and is starting to lose teeth, I'd recommend introducing this system – it shows it's the right time and will support their natural development.

The research goes on to show that by age 10, there are still 5 children in every 100 experiencing problems. So, not much progress is made with children who are left waiting for nature to take its' course.

POSSIBLE CAUSES

You may hear many reasons being put forward as possible causes of a bedwetting problem such as:

- the size of the bladder

- a urinary tract infection

- lack of hormones to concentrate urine

- something that runs in families

- stress or anxiety

Some children are referred to Enuresis Clinics by their GPs and, as a first step in the process, it is sensible to rule out the possibility of any infection which can easily be treated with antibiotics, or to identify the possibility of some other physiological cause for the problem.

Once it's been established that these possibilities do not play a part, the clinic will often suggest solutions such as using alarms in the bed which will wake the child once wetness is detected.

If alarms are not successful, children may be prescribed medication or drugs to concentrate their urine and even in extreme cases, will be offered anti-depressants.

Whilst some children will achieve a degree of success with these methods, in my experience, many of them revert to old habits within a short period and, in extreme cases, continue to wear protective pull-up pants at night until they are teenagers. Most children do eventually grow out of the bedwetting habit, but a small proportion will remain stuck in this pattern of behaviour and continue to wet the bed throughout their adult life. Without breaking this pattern of behaviour, the eventual effects are all too obvious.

In a minority of cases, there can be a sudden onset of bedwetting. If your child has been dry at night for several months or even years and starts having wet beds again, this can be caused by an emotional upset such as a change at home or stress with school work. This is usually temporary and not the same as an ongoing bedwetting problem. Most parents know their children and will be able to tell the difference, so if your gut feeling is that there is no real explanation for the bedwetting – go with your instincts but monitor the situation closely.

Neuro-psychologists now agree that there's a complex co-ordination that needs to take place between the nerves and the muscles of the bladder and more often than not, a delay in this happening is what holds children back.

New neural pathways or connections are needed to be made in the brain, in order to achieve night-time dryness and I'm going to show you how easy it can be to speed this process up.

CHAPTER 2

•

Understanding habits and behaviours

GETTING INTO THE HABIT

In the overwhelming majority of bedwetting cases, the cause is simply *habit*. Somehow over the years, your child got into a habit of wearing pull-up pants or similar absorbent protection and just never learnt how to stay dry all night. As simple as that.

And then you found yourselves caught in that 'catch 22' situation. Never quite confident enough to stop using absorbent pants (after all, think about the embarrassment an accident would cause if you were staying in a hotel) –but at the same time never quite giving your child's mind the opportunity to allow the neurological pathways to wire themselves up and create that 'auto-pilot'.

It's a common enough problem and in fact, it's the reason why more and more children are beginning to suffer from night-time bedwetting problems than ever before. Have you noticed how the supermarket shelves are increasingly stocking night-time 'pull-up' protective pants for teenagers up to the age of *15*?

A decade or so ago these just did not exist to the same extent. Make no mistake, the manufacturers are more than happy to keep on making these in all sorts of fancy designs and colours to keep your child happy.

But I believe, these may well be the cause of the problem, rather than a solution.

A quick survey of my bedwetting clients revealed that the average amount of money spent on protective night-time pants is £7 - £10 per week. Wow, just think how good you're going to feel when all that money can stay in your purse, rather than being thrown in the bin (quite literally!). And I wonder what you'll be spending it on........

PAST GENERATIONS

Quite a few of the bedwetting problems parents encounter today are as a result of lifestyle changes that have taken place in our society and the changes in our toilet training methods in general.

It's not uncommon nowadays to hear grandparents proudly announce that they never had problems toilet-training their young babies. And according to some - like my own mother – it was all over and done with by the age of 12 months! Of course, today's mums will roll their eyes up to the ceiling and take this piece of information with a pinch of salt.

But back in the days before disposable nappies had been invented, the incentive to get your baby dry and out of nappies was very much greater. Changing terry cloth nappies was hard work with hours of cleaning, boiling, sterilising and washing on a daily basis. Being a 'stay-at-home' mum was not so much a lifestyle choice but more of a necessity – someone had to do it.

And 'staying at home' also meant staying in one place for most of the day – making it very much easier to build up a routine for toilet training. Modern day mums are much more likely to be working outside the home, resulting in young children being ferried to and from nurseries or childminders.

Even our shopping habits have changed - most of us can spend several hours on a large supermarket visit rather than a quick 20 minute daily trip to the local shops, as was often the case years ago. Nowadays, it's a brave mother who's willing to chance her luck doing the shopping with a toddler in the throes of toilet-training. All this moving around, usually by car, makes dealing with 'accidents' that much harder.

Today's children have busy social lives and many start having sleepovers with friends at a much earlier age than they used to. So it's only natural that we do everything we possibly can to avoid those embarrassing accidents and encourage our children to continue wearing nappies or pull-ups for much longer.

The nappy manufacturers have done everything they can think of to make our lives easier and over the years they've improved the quality, fit and design to such an extent that your child no longer needs to even feel wet when they urinate. How comfortable can life get?

It's no wonder toilet training can become a bit of an uphill struggle for many parents – let's face it, life has to get a lot worse before it gets any better. Is there ever a good time to take off those nappies?

THE TRUE VALUE OF AN ACCIDENT

Avoiding accidents can mean missing out on valuable learning opportunities. Babies growing up in pre-disposable nappy days very quickly made a connection between urinating and feeling wet. Once this link was established, a second one was made – a relaxing of the bladder muscles and the release of urine.

And once you learn how to start something, you can quickly learn how to stop it. Constant repetition of a piece of behaviour – literally, your child weeing over and over again throughout the day – is what allows that vital mind / body connection to become more established. Having these experiences enables your child's mind to begin understanding changing behaviour.

Knowing this, it becomes easier to see why so many more children nowadays are struggling to master the art of bladder control. Not only are they missing out on the valuable learning opportunities that numerous toilet accidents throughout the day would have given them, but they're also missing out on the experience of feeling wet as the quality of nappies or pull-ups improves.

Our brains can be likened to a piece of plastic which moulds and adapts to fit the experiences in our environment. If your child never experiences the feeling of wetness when releasing urine from the bladder, those valuable connections in the brain cannot be made.

Of course, eventually all children will become toilet trained during the day – it just happens a little later nowadays than it used to. Getting dry at night then becomes the next hurdle to cross and many parents get stuck here – not knowing quite how to make this happen.

SELF-IMAGE

Your child's self-image plays a crucial role in literally predicting whether or not your child will be successful. Once the idea of being a bedwetter has established itself in your child's mind, it becomes a lot harder to change the pattern of behaviour.

Our behaviours will always match the image we have of ourselves and in this book, I'll be showing you how to ensure your child develops a positive self-image making success that much easier to achieve.

As scientists begin to discover and understand more about how our brains function, it's becoming increasingly clear that the best treatment for bedwetting is following a programme that encourages the child's mind to do one of two things:

either

> **get up when receiving a signal from the bladder and go to the bathroom**

or

> **stay asleep all night and hold on till the morning.**

I've devised this easy-to-read guide with activities and strategies for you and your child to follow over the course of 7 days to enable those vital connections to be established more quickly. We're going to speed up the body's natural processes.

The chances are that sooner or later, those vital connections will end up being made anyway – but why wait till your child is yet another year older? How many more sleepovers and school trips will be missed? How many more embarrassing moments will there be? And how much more washing will you tolerate?

With this system you'll be able to help your child beat this habit once and for all, in just a week.

Of course, you can get through it all in less than 7 days – most of the children who come to see me are dry on the first night after just one session. But I'm going to suggest that we take it a little more slowly and give your child's brain valuable thinking time before beginning to have those dry nights forever.

CREATING AN AUTO-PILOT

Conscious thinking uses different parts of the brain to unconscious learning so it's best to allow time for your child's brain to activate a deeper, more permanent intelligence.

After all, you're going to be asking your child to do things when they're half-asleep – in other words, not very conscious at all! The more deeply we can embed new patterns of behaviour on their subconscious minds, the easier it will be for them to operate on 'auto-pilot'.

Have you ever driven a car on a long journey and got to your destination unable to remember much about the driving part of it? That's because your conscious mind switched off for a while and started thinking about other things. Fortunately, the ability to drive has been imprinted on your subconscious mind so it was able to take over and do the job for you – your very own automatic pilot.

And you're going to be able to do exactly the same for your child – creating an automatic pilot that can register signals from the bladder, wake him up and steer him in the direction of the bathroom in the middle of the night. It's easier than you think.

CHAPTER THREE

•

Bedwetting, Hypnotherapy & NLP – a different solution to a familiar problem

WHAT'S THE BEST WAY TO STOP MY CHILD'S BEDWETTING HABIT?

Because of the stigma attached to bedwetting, most people start their search for help through the internet. Put "bedwetting" into any internet search engine and you will be given a number of different treatment options ranging from the use of electronic alarms,, medication to concentrate the flow of urine or even anti-depressants.

I know that each of these methods have differing levels of success and some parents will say that the alarms or medication have worked for their child. I can only say that in my experience of helping children with a bedwetting condition, these methods often only manage the problem in the short term rather than cure it for good and around 70% of children will go back to their old habits and behaviours after 2-3 months.

I helped one couple who had tried three different alarms, each of which had terrified their child before they consulted their family doctor who prescribed medication to reduce the flow of urine. This process went on for nearly two years before they brought their child to see me. Two years – that's a lot of wet sheets and pyjamas!!

WHAT'S THE ALTERNATIVE?

I believe the key to ending bedwetting once and for all is to encourage your child's mind and body to work more closely together. Children's minds are continually creating new connections called neural pathways, to accommodate new patterns of thinking and behaviour.

In my Hypnotherapy and NLP (Neuro-Linguistic Programming) practice, I've been seeing children with bedwetting problems regularly for the past 6 years. I have developed a quicker, safer and more natural alternative to changing night time habits for good. It doesn't involve any gadgets nor giving a child drugs - which has to be a good thing.

On average, nine out of ten children who come to see me for a session are dry that same night.

Following the session, I give them a series of visualisation exercises to do at home and a CD to listen to. It isn't always instant success and there may be one or two wet nights in the first couple of weeks but over a period of 3-4 weeks, a pattern of dry nights will start to establish itself.

HYPNOTHERAPY & NLP – IT'S CHILD PLAY

Whilst consulting a hypnotherapist may not be the solution that is uppermost in your mind to begin with, it is now becoming more widely accepted throughout the medical profession and many parents are referred to me by their family clinic and GP.

If the idea of hypnotising and reprogramming children's minds sounds a bit strange – fear not. During this stage of life, children's minds are like sponges absorbing all sorts of information naturally. In other words, they are being hypnotised all the time. You only have to observe a child's ability to gaze at the TV and recite the jingles back perfectly to see this in action.

That 'deeply relaxed state' is what we try to re-create during a session because, as you will have already witnessed when your child watches TV, information can be absorbed more deeply. In this instance, the information will be all about having dry beds forever.

Neuro-linguistic Programming, despite its' complicated name is really quite simple. NLP helps us to deal with what we think, what we say and what we do by breaking down our thought patterns and changing them for the better. Our thinking has a direct impact on our feelings and our behaviour.

Remember, your child's mind is being moulded and shaped by their environment all the time. In fact, your child spends many moments in a trance-like state every day, randomly absorbing all the messages around him. Some of these messages are good ones such as being praised for producing a good piece of homework - and others are not so helpful, such as having accidents and wetting the bed. Children quickly build up a picture of things they do well and things they do less well – and then go on to behave accordingly.

Techniques such as hypnotherapy and NLP are, in my opinion, under-utilised in the treatment of children but more parents are now turning to them as traditional methods fail to help their children.

As a result of the general lack of understanding about how these methods work, we are still more likely to prescribe unnecessary drugs and medication for our children, such as general anaesthetics to overcome dental phobias and drugs to reduce the flow of urine, rather than consider safer, more natural alternatives.

THE NORWEGIAN STUDY

In 2004, a study appeared in The Journal of the Norwegian Medical Association about using hypnotherapy to treat patients with chronic nocturnal enuresis. This study consisted of 12 boys ranging in age from 8 to 16.

All the boys had been diagnosed with primary nocturnal enuresis and four were also diagnosed with diurnal enuresis (daytime accidental urination). All 12 participants reported an average of 0 dry nights per week. The 12 participants also had a family history of bedwetting and had tried other forms of treatment such as bedwetting alarms and medication.

The boys had between 2 and 8 hypnotherapy sessions as part of the study and also practised self-hypnosis for one month after the sessions.

Two follow-ups were performed at 3 months and one year intervals. During both follow-ups, 9 out of the 12 participants reported 7 out of 7 dry nights per week. The researchers referred the 3 patients who continued to experience bedwetting to seek additional medical treatment.

The researchers concluded that hypnotherapy is an effective treatment for children diagnosed with nocturnal enuresis.

Source: Diseth, T.H. & Vandick, I.H. (2004)

CHAPTER FOUR

•

Getting started – how to use this book

HOW TO USE THIS BOOK

This book is for you and your child to use together. But, I do recommend that you read the book from start to finish *before* beginning to use this system with your child. You'll have a better idea of what's involved and how to implement it into your daily lives.

Before beginning, you'll need to discuss the plan of action with your child in detail explaining that soon they'll be free of this miserable habit – the embarrassment and wet beds.

You'll need to get your child's agreement by asking questions such as 'Does that sound ok to you?' or 'Are we going to do that?'.

It's possible to work through this book very quickly, but I'm going to advise that you take 7 days to allow your child's understanding to deepen. Mark a date on the calendar to indicate the day you will finally rid yourselves of this habit and begin a new life.

(If you prefer you can take up to 14 days to work through all the exercises, but make sure your child is doing at least one activity every day.)

GETTING STARTED

The activities that I've devised are a combination of listening, drawing and visualising. They all serve the same purpose and that is for you and your child to begin creating better pictures in your minds, as this will turn things around for you.

Up until now, your minds have been filled with images of wet sheets, extra laundry, embarrassment and feelings of failure. You probably both have a very good idea of how you don't want things to be and after a while it can become a lot harder to imagine a positive future. These activities are going to make it easier for you.

Having good pictures in our minds is an important step towards achieving success, for human beings are naturally drawn to the ideas in their minds. If the only thoughts and pictures your child has are of wet beds and failures, it's going to be a lot harder to achieve night-time dryness.

HYPNOTIC RECORDING

The first thing you will need to do is to DOWNLOAD a special recording from my website: www.stopbedwettingin7days.co.uk. This is available **free of charge** and your child will need to listen to this on a daily basis for at least a week. He'll need to start listening to this from Day 5 – so get prepared and download it onto an iPod or computer as soon as possible. If you prefer to have the recording on a CD, it's possible to order one of these through the website too.

Just 20 minutes long, this recording is filled with positive suggestions and visualisation exercises to help prepare your child's mind to be receptive to the idea of controlling his or her bladder at night without having to rely upon protective pants. It's best to provide a quiet time and place without interruptions at some point during the day for your child to do this.

Your child can listen to this once he is in bed at night, but during the first couple of days, it's good to include some 'daytime' listening too. But please, DO NOT play it whilst you are driving in the car or operating machinery – it's very relaxing and will encourage you to close your eyes!!

DRAWING ACTIVITIES

Some of the activities require your child to draw pictures - ensure you have a pad of A4 paper and some felt-tipped pens to hand. I have created some spaces within the book for these, but your child may wish to do some additional drawing. These drawing activities will help with that process of creating good ideas in your child's mind.

The activities should be preceded by a discussion between yourself and your child, so set aside 10-15 minutes for this. During a conversation, you'll be able to get your child thinking on the right track leaving them to complete the picture afterwards. Encourage your child to tell you about the picture in as many details as possible – this will ensure that positive ideas are cementing themselves in their minds.

EYES CLOSED / VISUALISATION ACTIVITIES

Other activities are visualisation techniques which are quite literally, eyes closed imagination games for you to play with your child. Although fairly simple to do, they do have a wonderful effect on helping people achieve their goals.

It's best to set aside 10-15 minutes for these and pick a time when you're unlikely to be interrupted.

Providing your child isn't too sleepy, incorporating these activities into your bedtime routine can be ideal.

KEEPING GOOD PICTURES IN MIND

Human beings are naturally goal-seeking and when I work with clients on self-improvement, one of the most important things I can tell them is "What you see, is what you get". As we think and speak, our minds are constantly making pictures, even if you're not aware of it. All throughout the day, your mind is doing this, whether you're thinking about phoning a friend, what to make for supper or what time you need to collect the children from school – little pictures will keep flashing through your mind.

We are magnetically drawn towards getting what we see and as with the drawing activities, the visualisation exercises will encourage your child's mind to focus on what they do want, rather than on what they don't want. As I've said before, it doesn't matter how badly you and your child want dry beds – if he or she can't imagine themselves in the future no longer needing to wear pants at night-time, they are not going to be able to do it.

These techniques are just like the ones used by top athletes and sports people. They know how much they can affect their performance. But they take it even one step further and 'mentally rehearse' themselves being even more successful if they want to improve and really become a winner. Runners see themselves running even faster, footballers see themselves scoring goal after goal. Your body cannot tell the difference between a vividly imagined experience and one that really happened.

Studies show that this kind of 'rehearsal' really does have a positive effect on the outcome. All sorts of magical wiring up takes place in the brain as you practise a scenario over and over and your child is going to be doing something very similar.

WHAT TO EXPECT

I've been seeing children for bedwetting sessions for nearly 6 years. During this time, the overwhelming majority of children – 9 out of 10 – are dry on the first night.

During the first week, dry nights continue but there may be a couple of wet ones too. However, over the subsequent three to four weeks the pattern of dry nights begins to establish itself with a wet night being a rarity.

It's going to be important to view any wet nights as 'one-off accidents' and not an indication that the system is not working. As already mentioned, these accidents provide valuable learning experiences for your child's mind and if your child has been wetting the bed at night for many *years*, it won't be surprising if it takes a few *days* to get the problem sorted out.

Imagine taking your car, storing it in a garage and locking it away for 8 or so years. Would you expect to be able to start it first time on taking it out again? Most probably not – you'd need to do a little tweaking and play around with a few wires and maybe even jumpstart it.

It will be a similar experience for getting your child dry at night and all the activities in this book are designed to 'jumpstart' the process of having dry nights forever.

JOSH'S STORY

Josh is aged 9 and his parents brought him along to see me as he was continuing to be wet every night. Having been referred to their local Enuresis Clinic, they had tried pretty much everything. Alarms did not seem to wake him up and when he was prescribed medication, this just made him urinate even more at night-time. He was wearing pull-ups every night and his parents also 'lifted' him just before they went to bed.

They had been trying a variety of methods for over two years with no success. Their doctor suggested they try hypnotherapy as a last resort.

In Josh's school, Year 6 pupils are taken away on a field trip for one week. Josh was beginning to worry – it was becoming more and more important for him to become dry at night, but there did not seem to be a solution.

Josh had two sessions with me – he carried out all the activities and listened to his CD. Rather unusually, Josh was not dry on the first night, nor on the second. By the third night, his parents were ready to abandon things but I persuaded them to stick with it. Josh's habit of night-time wetting was clearly deeply entrenched.

Much to everyone's relief, Josh had a dry night on the fifth night. He continued to have a run of dry nights for over a week before another wet night.

> *This turned out to be a 'one-off' and he went on to have another run of dry nights.*
>
> *Once in a while, he will have a wet night but overall he has managed to completely change his pattern of behaviour from wet to dry.*

I've highlighted this particular case for you because it was a bit trickier to solve. But despite struggling to begin with, it wasn't very long after that things just 'clicked' for Josh. 'Sticking with it' proved to be the key to success.

Josh's mum emailed me recently:

"Josh has had a further 6 dry nights in a row and we are all ecstatic. On behalf of all of us, I want to say how grateful we are. Josh seems to be changing too – he seems happier and less moody. It's only now we can see what effect this had on all of us especially Josh – he was becoming so downbeat.

Josh has asked me to say 'I am very happy it has worked and thank you very much'."

CHAPTER FIVE

•

The Final Countdown

BEFORE YOU BEGIN

Before beginning this system, it's worth taking a look at your child's environment and checking if it's possible to make achieving success that little bit easier.

First of all, here are some things you will need:

- Sheets of A4 paper

- Felt-tipped pens

- A couple of ordinary party balloons

- Notebook for recording success

- Downloadable audio recording

PICK YOUR MOMENT

Choosing the right moment to introduce this system to your child can mean the difference between success and failure. Pick your moment carefully. Is your child ready to tackle this problem? Do they recognise that it is something that can be dealt with? Do they have a desire to change?

It's not a good idea to pick a week that you know is going to be a particularly busy one with school exams for example. Likewise if you plan to be away from home for a couple of nights, it may disrupt the continuity of the programme.

The school holidays may prove to be the best time for your child, but for others the lack of routine and late nights may cause more problems. You'll know best which week will be right for you – but do plan ahead.

ELECTRICAL EQUIPMENT

I am not a great fan of TVs and computers in children's bedrooms. Nowadays it's easy to become overloaded with electrical gadgets if we include clock radios, mobile phones, TVs, Playstations, computers and Blackberries.

Scientific experts are beginning to agree that sleeping in an electromagnetic field does not aid restful sleep. I would recommend clearing the 'energy space' in your child's bedroom as much as possible by removing as many electrical items as you can.

The visualisation techniques in this book are designed to help your child's brain make new neural connections and wire itself up in a different way. This will be taking place as your child sleeps and dreams – the less interference the better. Playing exciting computer games or watching TV for a short while before going sleep will add to the confusion in your child's mind just at the moment when it will be needed the most.

TOO LIGHT OR TOO DARK?

Some children who come to see me will often reveal in a session that they "would go to the bathroom at night, only it's too dark". Would this apply to your situation?

Have a check that the route to the bathroom is well lit. However, whilst it's important to have light on the outside, I would recommend having less light inside the bedroom. Experts do agree that night-lights are best switched off as your child begins to grow up. Your child will experience a deeper, better quality sleep if the room is dark and this alone may ensure a dry night.

CLUTTER

Your child is going to be asked to get out of bed and find the route to the bathroom in the middle of the night, should he feel the need to use the toilet. Before doing this, it's worth ensuring that the floor space is completely clear.

Left-over jigsaw puzzles, games, toys and piles of dirty clothes that can be tripped over will not add to your child's confidence about his ability to make it to the bathroom in the dark.

BATHROOM

And what about the bathroom or toilet? One child who came to see me admitted that he was scared to go to the loo at night because of 'the black toilet seat'. It wasn't so much a case of not wanting to admit it to his mother sooner – it really hadn't occurred to him until he started talking to me about it. It's worth taking the time to make the bathroom as child-friendly as possible.

Position as many items as possible at child-height – eg. mirrors, towel rails, soap and even small wash-hand basins if possible.

Allowing your child to choose some of the accessories, such as colourful handtowels will help your child to feel that this space belongs as much to him as to the adults in the house.

CHANGING DRINKING HABITS

There's conflicting advice regarding how many drinks a child who is trying to stop bedwetting, should or shouldn't have each day.

Some experts recommend children drink more water during the day to allow the bladder to stretch and get used to accommodating more liquid at night. Others will recommend restricting drinks and certainly none at all after about 4.30pm in the afternoon.

But then again, some feel that constipation may be one of the reasons for bedwetting – and they would advocate increasing fluids throughout the day.

It's no wonder some parents feel confused.

Personally, I'm not in favour of restricting fluids in young children and certainly not on hot summer days. I feel common-sense should prevail – if your child is thirsty, he or she should be able to have a drink.

However, some of the children who have followed my programme noticed that they were more likely to have a wet bed if they'd had too many sugary, fizzy drinks (including fruit juices) or caffeinated drinks (such as cola, chocolate, tea or coffee) the day before. So, my advice would be 'keep it simple' – let's stick to plain water wherever possible but don't make a big deal of it.

CHANGING EATING HABITS

Certain foods can also have an effect on your child's bladder – the main culprits being wheat and dairy foods. And be aware of the diuretic effect of certain fruits such as strawberries and the artificial sweeteners that are put into so many of children's foods. Read more about these on my website.

STAYING POSITIVE

It's important to remain encouraging and enthusiastic throughout this period. Remember, the more confident you can appear, the more likely your child is to be successful.

Praise your child regularly and be sympathetic if they have an accident one night. Remind your child that sticking to the exercises will ensure that they have dry nights forever.

DEALING WITH ACCIDENTS

It is possible that your child will be dry *every* night from Day 7, but it's probably unlikely. Planning in advance will make any accidents much easier to deal with. Have plenty of spare sheets and bedding as well as a plastic protective cover for the mattress.

Consider making up the bed with two layers of sheets and placing an absorbent mat or pad in between these layers. If your child does wet the bed in the middle of the night, you'll be able to quickly remove the top sheet together with the absorbent pad, giving you a ready-made dry bed for him or her to climb into quickly. This will minimise night-time disruptions.

CHAPTER SIX

•

The Three Golden Rules

THE THREE GOLDEN RULES

There are just 3 simple rules that I'm going to ask you follow to give your child the best possible chance of success.

<u>RULE NUMBER ONE</u>

No protective pull-up pants or nappies ever again.

Using this system, you'll develop the confidence to clear out the cupboards and rid yourselves of those protective pants that cost a fortune and harm the environment.

By Day 7 of this programme your task will be to throw them all in the bin. It's important to stick to this rule. Don't be tempted to keep some back 'just in case', as you'll be programming your child's mind for failure rather than success.

However, it is acceptable to use a protective mattress cover in case of accidents. In the meantime, just think how much money you will be saving by never having to buy nappies or protective pants again. Calculate this figure and write it here ....

RULE NUMBER TWO

No lifting.

It's common to receive advice about 'lifting'. This involves waking up your child just as you are going to bed and 'encouraging' them to have one last wee before continuing with the rest of the night's sleep.

On the face of it, sounds like a good idea but not only is it an unpleasant experience for your child (would you like to be woken in the middle of the night and dragged off to the loo?), but you are actively encouraging your child to wee in the night.

It's important to remember what the real goal of this exercise is. Your goal is to help your child achieve night time dryness. By lifting, you are in fact *training* your child to not only release urine when half asleep, but to also develop a need to go to the toilet in the middle of the night. However well intentioned, it's not helpful to the process so let's leave it out.

RULE NUMBER THREE

No Reward Systems

This rule may seem a bit strange as we've become so accustomed to developing reward systems for our children to encourage them to do almost anything. Automatically, we assume that if we want to create a change in behaviour it's not going to be possible without the involvement of star charts, sweeties or trips out.

I'm going to suggest a slightly different approach. It is important to record moments of success and I've provided a special diary for tracking progress further on.

Psychological studies have shown that behaviour that gets measured or observed often improves spontaneously. The attention to detail adds momentum to the process making it easier to achieve our goals.

Combining rewards or treats with a goal-oriented programme however, can just lead to confusion. There's proof that the most helpful way to get your child motivated and successful is to focus on the goal itself – in this case, 'dry beds forever', rather than the 'prize' that will be awarded as a result of it.   Remember, your child needs to channel all of his brainpower into making that vital connection between the bladder, muscles and the mind – it's best not to create distractions with promises of sweets or trips out to theme parks – you'll actually be making it harder for your child to succeed.

The 3 golden rules are:

1. **No pull-ups, nappies or protection at night.**

2. **No lifting.**

3. **No reward systems.**

This will be your new routine from Day 7 of the programme. In the meantime, if you're still using pull-ups keep doing so until the instructions tell you to stop.

CHAPTER SEVEN

•

All About Me

Day One

ALL ABOUT ME

Welcome to the first day of this life-changing programme for your child. Today there two activities for you and your child to complete:

Building a positive self-image

Always... Sometimes...... Never

Set aside plenty of time (15 – 20 minutes) to discuss the activities and brainstorm together, perhaps making a few notes first. These activities are designed to put your child into the right frame of mind for making this big change in their lives.

BUILDING A POSITIVE SELF-IMAGE

It's not unusual for children who have a history of wetting their beds at night, to have a poor self-image. This is especially so if the problem has continued for many years.

However hard parents may have tried to minimise the negative impact, it won't have escaped the child's attention that their lives are full of wet, smelly pants or sheets and that they can't quite do what other children can do – such as have sleepovers easily with their friends.

If other methods to solve the bedwetting problem, such as the use of alarms, medication or lifting have also been tried with no success, this will just add to the child's perception of themselves as a failure.

It's really important to reinforce your child's perception of himself as a good, worthwhile, confident and successful person. The more you can build up this image, the more likely your child is to be successful. The pictures we create in our minds with our imaginations play a very big part in determining what happens in our lives.

ACTIVITY 1 - All About me

Step 1:

Complete the details below. Depending on your child's age and writing abilities, this section may be completed by yourself or your child, whichever is easier. Take 15 minutes or so to discuss your child's strengths.

Some things about me:

My name is . . . .

My age is . . . .

My favourite colour is . . . .

My favourite food is. . . . .

My friends' names are . . . .

Now make a list of things that your child is good at or found easy to learn – for example: colouring pictures, taking care of a pet, jumping on the spot – these can be as varied and random as you like and as simple or complicated as you'd like.

Things I am good at

. . . .

. . . .

. . . .

. . . .

. . . .

. . . .

. . . .

. . . .

Step 2:

Now ask your child to list activities that they struggled with initially, but eventually mastered –things that were a little trickier to learn, such as riding a bike, swimming, writing their name or learning times tables.

> ### Things I had to practise before I became successful:
>
> . . . .
>
> . . . .
>
> . . . .
>
> . . . .
>
> . . . .
>
> . . . .
>
> . . . .

Remind your child:

Once upon a time, he or she couldn't walk and couldn't talk, or even feed themselves, but gradually over time these were new things that they learnt and can now do quite easily.

And having dry beds is just one more of those things that they will easily learn.

ACTIVITY 2 – Always, Sometimes, Never

It's interesting how easy it is to get locked into the idea of failure. Once an idea is firmly established in the mind (eg. my child still wets the bed at night), we unconsciously seek out evidence to support this idea. In other words, it will become so easy to remember all those accidents and the wet sheets that needed washing, that we'll cancel out any moments of success.

In this activity, I'm going to ask you to consider the following questions:

*Is your child **always** wet at night?*

*Does he or she **sometimes** have a dry night?*

*Has he or she **never** had a dry night?*

I always ask these questions when parents come to see me with their children. It's very common for them to reply "Well, there was one dry night when we stayed at Grandma's at Christmas...... but that doesn't count.... as we all went to bed so late."

Well – it does count! It very much counts. These odd random moments of dryness are very important...... concrete proof or evidence to your child that they can be dry.... they do have the ability to remain dry throughout the night, they just need a little more practise, that's all.

Fill in the box on the next page and record any successes in relation to dry beds that your child has had in the past. Sometimes a stay at Grandma's or at a friend's house has resulted in a dry night.

If your child has really never had a dry night, is there any other 'evidence' that you can remember that suggests a degree of success – eg. staying dry till 5am in the morning or not being 'lifted' on another occasion. It's important to demonstrate to your child that the same thing doesn't always happen every night. Different things do happen sometimes – they are not locked into a set pattern of behaviour each and every night.

When have I been dry?

. . . .

. . . .

. . . .

. . . .

. . . .

. . . .

. . . .

. . . .

Use this as evidence to demonstrate to your child that they can be successful in achieving this on a permanent basis.

CHAPTER EIGHT

•

My New Future

Day Two

MY NEW FUTURE

Spend a few moments reviewing and discussing the exercises from yesterday. Perhaps your child will have thought of a few more ideas overnight to add in to their lists.

There are two new activities for you today:

My New Future – Step 1

My New Future – Step 2

MY NEW FUTURE – STEP 1

Today, I'd like you to invite your child to take a glimpse into the future. That wonderful future when everything is just the way he or she would like it to be.............. waking up each morning with a dry bed. Begin by asking:

What will you see?

What will you feel?

What will you hear?

Ask your child to draw a picture on the next page showing how fantastic waking up in the morning will be. This is an important step towards getting him or her to be able to visualise a new future clearly. Without this, it will be much harder for them to achieve success.

Include as much information as possible – the bed with dry sheets, the time on the clock and perhaps even the weather outside.

Ask your child to remember to include themselves in the picture .... with a big smile on his or her face. They can add in other people, perhaps having them speaking some words. Encourage your child to write some words underneath the picture.

Note: if your child is really reluctant to draw pictures, you can ask them to describe the scene in detail to you and make notes instead. The aim of the exercise is to get as much detail as possible recorded – remember to answer the questions at the beginning of the exercise.

MY NEW FUTURE LOOKS LIKE THIS:

Complete this sentence: *When I have dry beds in the morning, this is what I will see, hear and feel:*

....

....

....

MY NEW FUTURE – STEP 2

Now take a few moments to encourage your child to think about what else will happen as a result of having dry beds. Ask the following questions:

As well as having a dry bed, what else will change in your life? Will it change the way you feel?

And what about the other people around you? How will they feel? Imagine who else will be there first thing in the morning and the kind of things that they might say.

Imagine yourself being successful and having dry beds - will it mean you can start to do different things, like have sleepovers with friends? Will it mean you can go on holidays and school trips more easily?

What's the very best thing that will happen to you when you are dry at night?

What will you see?

What will you hear?

What will you feel?

Complete this sentence: When I have dry beds it will mean

that ....

....

Ask your child to pick two examples and draw pictures below to show how much better things will look.

CHAPTER NINE

•

Mind over body

Day Three

MIND OVER BODY

Welcome to Day 3 of the programme – progress is being made.

As before, take a few moments to discuss and review the ideas that came up for you and your child in the previous activities. Talking will help reinforce ideas in your child's mind.

There are FOUR new activities for you to cover today:

How My Body Works

Controlling Muscles

Water Balloon

Gate Visualisation

As there are four activities for you to do today, I'm going to suggest splitting them into 2 separate sessions, as I've indicated above.

HOW MY BODY WORKS

It's important for your child to have a better understanding of how the body works and what it's going to be asked to do. Explain to your child that the mind and body are connected and have a conversation with each other throughout the day.

Sometimes our bodies tell us what to do and sometimes we tell our bodies what to do.

Your body tells you:

- If you're too hot - *you might want to take your jumper off*

- If you're too cold - *you'll feel like putting a jumper on*

- If you're hungry - *your tummy will start to rumble*

- If you're thirsty - *your mouth will feel dry*

- If you're tired - *you'll start yawning*

And then there are those other times when you tell your body to do things:

- You tell it to run
- You tell it to jump
- You tell it to speak out loud
- You tell it to pick up a pencil and write

And telling your body to *hang on and walk* to the bathroom to use the toilet if you need to, is just one more of those things you'll be able to teach it to do.

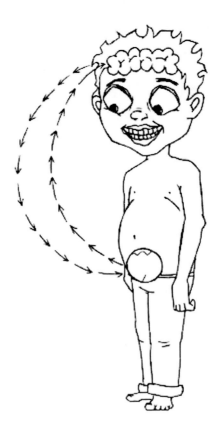

CONTROLLING MUSCLES

The bladder is a pouch or bag made of muscle that opens and closes as it tenses and relaxes.

Our bodies are full of muscles that can do this – we have them in our arms and legs, fingers and toes and we can tell them exactly what to do. We tell the muscles in our bodies to do things all the time.

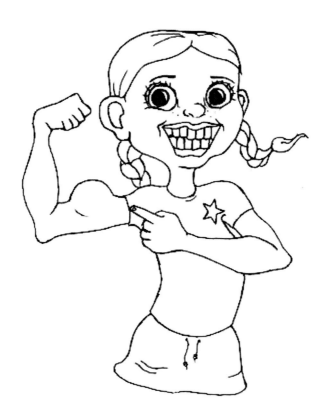

Take a few moments, find a quiet space to sit or lie down with your child and discover what I mean as you play this game with your child.

Hands: *Clench each fist (one at a time) for three seconds and then relax it for three seconds.*

Arms: *Bend each elbow so the wrist nearly touches the shoulder (one at a time) and hold for 3 seconds, then relax each arm for 3 seconds.*

Legs: *Point the toes and straighten the leg, pushing the knee down, so both the calf and thigh muscles tighten for 3 seconds, then relax this leg for 3 seconds. Repeat with the other leg.*

Shoulders: *Pull the shoulders up to the ears (or as close as they can get) and hold for 3 seconds, then relax for a further 3 seconds.*

Eyes: *Scrunch up the eyes so that they are tightly shut for 3 seconds. Then relax the eyes, but keep them shut for at least 3 seconds.*

And in just the same way, it's possible to control the bladder – opening it and closing it as and when needed. The muscles act like a 'gate' on the bladder.

Try this experiment and you'll see what I mean.

Handy tip: trying this in the bath may be the best place!!

WATER BALLOON EXPERIMENT

1. Take an ordinary party balloon (a round one is best) and attach it to the end of a cold water tap.

2. Switch the tap on slowly and watch as the water begins to fill the balloon. Keep going until it's a bit bigger than a tennis ball. Switch the water off.

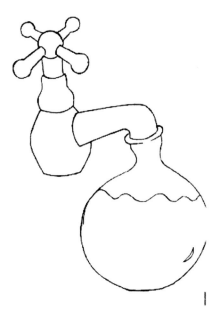

3. Now, very carefully take the balloon off the tap and squeeze the open end between your thumb and one of your fingers, to make sure the water can't come out.

4. Turn the balloon upside down over the sink. This is similar to how your bladder looks. Slowly, begin to relax your fingers slightly and allow some water to begin trickling out of the end. This is just how water comes out of your bladder when you go to the toilet.

5. Now let's see if we can stop this flow. Squeeze your fingers tight once more and you'll discover that you can easily stop the water coming out.

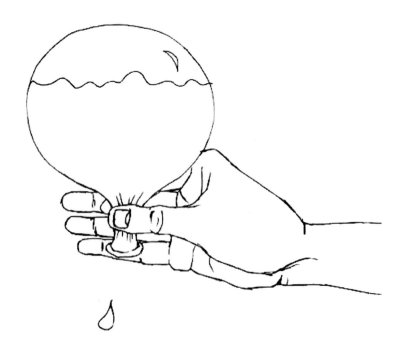

6. Relax your fingers a little once more and let a bit more water out.

7. And then squeeze them tightly shut to stop the flow once more.

This is exactly how your muscles work – squeezing tight to hold urine in the bladder and relaxing to let it out – just like opening and closing a gate.

You can practise this exercise again, if you want to. Keeping this gate tightly closed is just what your body needs to learn to do at night to help you keep your bed dry.

GATE VISUALISATION

Now we know how the muscles in our body open and close around the bladder just like a gate, we're going to take a closer look at your child's 'gate'. Everyone's is different and I wonder what his or hers will look like.

Try this activity.

---

1. *Settle yourselves down somewhere comfortable. Ask your child to close his eyes and just take a few moments to visualise the gate to his bladder. Pause for a few moments to give your child time to do this.*

2. *Encourage him to describe it clearly to you*

    ☐ *what colour is it?*
    ☐ *how does it open?*
    ☐ *does it have a lock or bolt on it?*
    ☐ *is the lock tightly shut right now?*

3. *Ask your child to tell you what needs to be done to make sure this gate is firmly shut at night. (Allow your child's imagination to take over here – some children invent gatekeepers, or put extra big locks on)..*

Now ask your child to draw a picture of this gate
here.............

My gate looks like this!!

CHAPTER TEN

•

Pump up the volume!

Day Four

PUMP UP THE VOLUME

Welcome to Day 4 – you're halfway through the programme now.

Take some time to review and chat about the exercises from the previous days. If you feel there is any confusion or lack of understanding, you'll be able to remind your child that each day they are getting closer and closer to achieving their goal – Dry Nights Forever!

There are two more exercises to carry out today:

Volume Control Exercise

Saying What you Want

Note: from tomorrow your child will need to start listening to the Hypnotic Recording – Dry Beds Now. If you haven't done so already, DOWNLOAD it from my website now – www.stopbedwettingin7days.co.uk . – it's free of charge and getting it now will mean that you'll have it to hand when you need it.

VOLUME CONTROL EXERCISE

Some nights it isn't going to be possible to wait until morning to visit the toilet - some nights your child may need to get up and go to the loo. We already know this.

But in the past, your child's mind and body just haven't been communicating well enough to enable this to happen. Your child has remained in bed and you've dealt with the consequences in the morning.

During the day, your child gets messages from the bladder many times. A little voice gets heard in the mind – *"need to go to the toilet"* – and your child responds by walking to the bathroom and successfully dealing with the situation. Point this out to your child and ask them to pay specific attention to what receiving this message feels like, for the next few days.

During the night your child is asleep. So when that little voice pipes up – *"need to go to the toilet"* – it doesn't get heard.

There's a very simple solution to this. Let's turn the volume UP.

Take a few moments to run through this activity with your child. Begin by explaining to your child that he hears that little voice inside his head many times a day. It not only speaks up when it needs to go to the loo, but it's the same voice that says

"hmm, I'm hungry, I fancy a biscuit"

"I'm feeling hot – I want to take my jumper off"

"I wonder what's on television"

and getting it to speak a little louder at night time, is just one of those things that can easily be done.

1. *Ask your child to think of a favourite piece of music. This could be a song that they really like, the theme tune to a TV programme or even the 'Happy Birthday' song.*

2. *Ask them to tell you what it is and to just let themselves hear that music playing in their imaginations – ie. not out loud. Keep playing this music for a few moments.*

3. *Now it's time for a bit of fun. Get your child to play around with the volume by saying "I wonder if you can make it just a little bit quieter? And a little bit quieter still?" Pause here for a few moments to allow your child to do this.*

4. *And now you can turn the volume up by saying "And how about making it louder? .... And a bit more?......... I wonder if you can make it so loud that it would wake the baby/frighten the dog (or similar)". Again pause for a few moments to allow your child to do this. It's usual to see an intense look of concentration accompanied by a few giggles as they get the hang of this.*

5. *Take a few more moments to play around turning the volume back down so it's nice and quiet and up, up, up so it's really loud once more.*

THE VOLUME CONTROL

We don't know what your child's volume control looks like. Each one of us has a control that looks slightly different.

Point out to your child some of the different controls that can be found around the house – for example: the light switch that flicks on and off, or maybe it's a dimmer that rotates around. Some switches are dials, others are levers and some have buttons like the controls for the television.

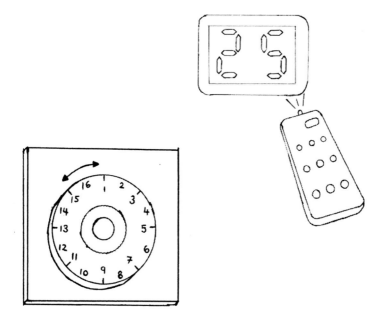

1. *Ask your child to close his eyes for a few moments to take a really good look at the volume control that controls the sounds inside his mind.*

2. *What colour is it? How about the shape – is it round, square or long? Does it have a dial or a button?*

3. *How does he know which setting it's on – does it have numbers 1-10 or higher? Or does it say Low-Medium-High?*

4. *Ask your child to play around with the volume setting – can they turn it right down low? And then right up high, so it's very much louder?*

Ask your child to draw a picture of his very own special volume control here:

This is my volume control!

Now that we know what that all important volume control looks like, your child will be able to easily programme it each night before going to sleep.

AUTOMATIC PILOT

We've all had situations where we've had to get up extra specially early in the morning – perhaps to go off on holiday and catch an early morning flight.

Have you ever set the alarm clock for some crazy time like 4am, worried that you might oversleep but somehow miraculously found yourself automatically waking up five minutes before the alarm goes off?

It's a strange feeling, isn't it?   People often wonder why that happens - in reality, not only do we set the alarm clock but we also programme our subconscious minds to wake us up as we're doing it. So, when we wake up early, we're literally operating on 'automatic pilot'.

In just the same way, your child can programme his very own 'automatic pilot' to wake himself up when he receives that signal from his bladder.

ADJUSTING THE VOLUME

1. *Ask your child to close his eyes and see in his imagination the volume control for the bladder – this may look a little different to the one that was controlling the music – check with your child and ask him to describe it once more.*

2. *What is the control set at? Is it set on high? Or is it set on low? Should it be adjusted?*

3. *Pause for a few moments here to allow your child to make whatever adjustments he or she feels are necessary to set this volume control on a loud enough setting to wake him up during the night, should he need to visit the toilet.*

Every evening just before settling down for the night, your child will need to run through this activity and just check the control is set at the right level.

WHAT YOU <u>SAY</u> IS WHAT YOU <u>SEE</u>

As we've already discovered, our minds are constantly making pictures in response to the words that come into our minds. If I ask you now NOT to think of a piece of chocolate cake, there'll be no prizes for guessing what picture comes straight into your mind. Whether you wanted to or not, chocolate cake is what you saw.

Your mind had no option but to do this, as there's no picture it can make for the word *'not'* – so you got left with precisely what you didn't want to see.

That's why it's going to be really important to be conscious of the words that you speak to your child whilst working through this programme. The emphasis is going to be on having 'dry beds' rather than 'not having wet beds'.

We are magnetically drawn towards the pictures we make in our imaginations – so it's important to always be making good ones.

SAYING WHAT YOU WANT

Keeping in mind the importance of thinking and saying what it is we DO want to happen, rather than what we DON'T want to happen, ask your child to spend a few moments each evening saying the following phrases out loud just before going to bed each night.

These phrases will be the equivalent of setting that alarm clock – your child's automatic pilot:

"While I'm sleeping tonight bladder, if you start filling up – be sure to send a really loud message to my brain to let me know".

"Turn the volume up really loud, so that I can hear you".

"And remember to keep the gate shut until you wake me up, so I can get up out of my dry bed and walk to the bathroom in time."

Saying these phrases slowly, deliberately and out loud will send a flow of energy, almost like a crackle of electricity, down a particular neural pathway creating that vital link between mind and body.

Handy Tip : Either you or your child can copy these sentences out onto sticky post-it notes and stick them on the wall next to the bed. Each evening, just before tucking down to sleep, your child will be able to say them out loud once more.

CHAPTER ELEVEN

•

Programming your Sat-Nav

Day Five

PROGRAMMING YOUR SAT-NAV

Welcome to Day 5. Praise your child for having done really well to get this far. There are not too many days to go now. Remind him that in just a couple of days, he'll be enjoying the benefits of having those 'dry nights'.

As your programme progresses and the activities begin to build up, you may want to review yesterday's at a different time to introducing the new ones today. There is just one visualisation exercise to carry out today and your child will need to start listening to the Hypnotic Recording – "Dry Beds Now!!" – which you can get free from my website at *www.stopbedwettingin7days.co.uk*.

Have you downloaded your copy yet?

Today's activities are:

Sat Nav Programming

Listening to Hypnotic Recording

SAT- NAV PROGRAMMING

Most of us wouldn't set off on a long journey without putting our destination into our satellite navigation systems, printing off directions from the internet or checking a map. Only when we have a pretty good idea of where we're heading and how to get there, do we set off.

Expecting your child to get up in the middle of the night, in the dark and visit the bathroom in a semi-conscious state is a bit like playing 'Blind-man's Buff' at a children's party. It's no wonder most kids opt to stay in bed and not venture out. So how can we give your child a map to navigate by?

Step One

Begin by starting this activity during the daytime when there is some light and it is a little less daunting. After the first couple of attempts, you can close the bedroom curtains to make it more realistic. It's really important to reinforce your child's perception of himself as someone who can easily get up and walk to the bathroom at night, should they need to. The more this is 'rehearsed', the more likely your child is to be successful.

1. *Ask your child to climb into bed and snuggle down under the covers, as if going to sleep at night.*

2. *Next, ask him/her to imagine that they've just received the signal that it's time to go to the loo. Ask them to turn the volume up and really hear that voice inside their head.*

3. *Guide your child out of bed and walk slowly together along the route to the bathroom.*

4. *As you're walking along describe the route out loud: eg. turn left, straight along for six steps, out of the door, into the hallway, eight steps past the cupboard and Mum and Dad's bedroom, a few more steps and into the bathroom. Describe the route exactly as you see it.*

5. *Repeat this process several more times, until your child knows it off by heart and can say it out loud by themselves.*

Step Two

Having established the best route for your child to use at night time, it's time to ensure that this becomes firmly imprinted on your child's mind by rehearsing it over and over again. This way, their personal "sat-nav" system is fully programmed.

Remember, if your child needs to go to the loo during the night, he or she will only be semi-conscious – this needs to be something they can do without thinking.

---

1. *Ask your child to lay down on the bed once more and close their eyes. Once again, ask them to imagine that they've just received the signal (ie. heard that very loud voice) from their bladder that they need to go to the loo.*

2. *This time, they can allow themselves to just picture themselves walking to the bathroom in their imagination. They won't need to do it 'for real', but your child will need to describe the route to the bathroom out loud a couple of times over. As you listen to this, check that their details are correct.*

---

3. *Now they'll be ready to just run through the scenario in their minds without saying anything at all. Repeat this several times over.*

Remember – our bodies can't tell the difference between a real and an imagined event. This is a very clever way of 'rehearsing' the future, tricking your body into believing that you have done this before - making it all the easier to do it 'for real' when the time comes.

LISTENING TO THE AUDIO RECORDING

Have you downloaded your FREE audio recording from my website yet?

www.stopbedwettingin7days.co.uk

The audio recording lasts around twenty minutes. Your child will need to have a quiet place to listen to this. It's filled with positive messages which will reinforce all the work we've done so far.

It can be listened to once your child is in bed, in place of a bedtime story. However, as it's possible they will drift off to sleep whilst listening to it, I'd recommend giving them the opportunity to listen to it earlier in the day too. It's not necessary to be lying down with eyes closed – if your child is having a quiet moment playing with puzzles for example, you can have the recording playing in the background.

Please DO NOT play it whilst you are driving in the car or operating machinery. It's very relaxing!!

Before your child goes to sleep tonight, I recommend running through this short list of activities.

TONIGHT'S BEDTIME CHECKLIST

- Visualise gate on bladder and close it tight. ☐

- Set volume control on HIGH. ☐

- Speak 'auto-pilot phrases' out loud. ☐

- Programme Sat Nav ☐

- Listen to audio recording. ☐

CHAPTER TWELVE

•

Nearly There

Day Six

NEARLY THERE – JUST SOME LAST MINUTE PREPARATIONS!!

As you and your child reach the final day of preparation for your new life of "DRY BEDS FOREVER", now is the time to take a few moments to just check if there are any last minute doubts, worries or niggles that could hold your child back. Tonight, you'll be repeating several of the activities and leaving those protective pull-up pants or nappies behind forever. The time for collecting up every last one in the house and disposing of them for good is not very far away.

First of all, it's important to check that each and every 'part' of you and your child is happy with the decision to move forward in this way. It's common to feel in 'two minds' about certain things because two minds is exactly what we have – our conscious mind and our subconscious mind. It's easy to feel as if we know what we want to achieve on the outside but sometimes, our insides can almost 'sabotage' our attempts.

How many of us adults want to lose weight but on the other hand, also really fancy that extra piece of chocolate cake? Have you ever wanted to get fit and go to the gym, but on the other hand really wanted to stay on the sofa and watch a movie?

The same goes for our children. Perhaps on the one hand they really want to spend time doing their school homework to get good marks, but on the other hand they also want to spend time playing a video game or watching TV.

Success becomes much harder to achieve when there's a little bit of an internal struggle going on. Take a few moments now to discuss any last doubts or worries that both of you may be having.

Perhaps you're really looking forward to having dry nights forever with no more pull-ups, but on the other hand you also want to ensure the bed sheets are dry. On the one hand, it would be nice to save lots of money from not having to buy protective pants or pull-ups but, on the other hand, will the money be spent on lots of extra washing of wet sheets?

Perhaps your child is looking forward to having sleepovers with their friends, but, on the other hand, the safety and security of home where they can keep their pull-ups on is also appealing?

All of these negative feelings are serving a purpose – they are trying to protect you and your child and their intention is good. Even though it feels as if you are being pulled in two different directions, both sides only want the best for you. However, those feelings can have a sabotaging effect and hold you back from what you'd really like to achieve. Always keep in mind your ultimate goal – what would you really like to have happen? What is your dream?

ACHIEVING AGREEMENT

1. Take a few moments to identify any last minute worrying beliefs that you or your child may have. You may want to discuss these issues and write them down on a piece of paper.

2. Once you have done this, place your hands out in front of you with your palms facing up to the ceiling. Imagine the part that wants dry beds in your right hand and the other part, the bit that sometimes holds you back, in your left.

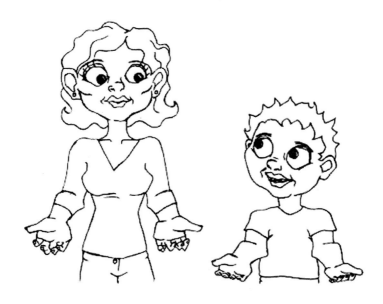

3. *As you look at each hand in turn, ask the part what its' positive intention is for you. Continue asking each part until it becomes increasingly obvious that they both want the same thing for you – namely, dry beds, success and happiness.*

4. *Keep running through this process, even if it feels a little strange to begin with. Doing this will create changes in your confidence and self-belief.*

5. *Imagine a new 'super-part' emerging in the space between your hands. A 'super-part' that has the resources to keep both of those other parts happy and still create success for you. As you look down into this space, you may want to give it a colour – a special colour - a colour that feels right for you.*

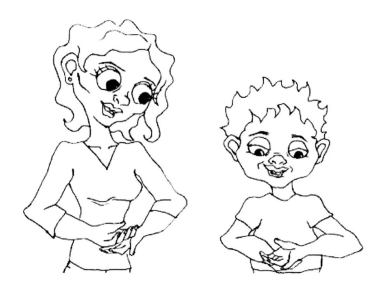

6. *Now moving quickly, bring your hands together and allow those two separate parts to merge with the super-part and become one.*

7. *Raise your hands up to your chest and bring them in, allowing this new 'super' part to become fully absorbed and integrated as a new bit of you.*

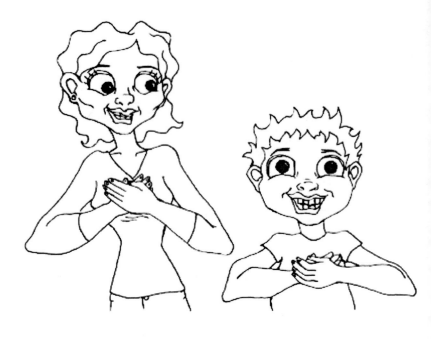

8. Close your eyes and enjoy this feeling of having every bit of your body in agreement about the kind of future you'll have.

As you practise this technique, you'll find all those feelings of internal conflict begin to simply disappear. You and your child both have a goal in mind – dry beds forever – and as all those parts line up in agreement, you'll find it easier to achieve just that.

TONIGHT'S BEDTIME CHECKLIST

- Visualise gate on bladder and close it tight. ☐

- Set volume control on HIGH. ☐

- Speak 'auto-pilot phrases' out loud. ☐

- Programme Sat Nav ☐

- Listen to audio recording. ☐

CHAPTER THIRTEEN

•

Dry Nights Forever

Day Seven

DRY NIGHTS FOREVER

Well done – you've reached the end of the programme and the beginning of that new future.

Each day for the next week, it's going to be important for your child to continue to listen to the Hypnotic Recording which you've downloaded.

Additionally, there'll be that bedtime checklist of activities to run through.

NO MORE PROTECTIVE NIGHT-TIME PANTS

You have now reached the moment where you can throw out those nappies, pull-ups, pads, liners, alarms – whatever it is you were using to keep the bed dry at night. As your child's mind and body start to work closer together now than ever before, you'll discover that you no longer have a need for them.

Spend some time with your child and hunt through your cupboards, under the beds and even in the garage, to track down every last pull-up in the house. Bundle them all together in a plastic sack and throw them as far away as possible – certainly not in the house!!

Really enjoy this moment together - this is an important step forward in your child's development and the more confident you can be as you do this, the more confident your child will feel.

I am often asked by clients "Should I keep a couple of pull-ups just in case?". As tempting as this will be, I would recommend that you do not do this. "Just in case" or "for emergencies" really means "in case this doesn't work" and you'll be programming your mind to do just that – fail. Programme your mind for success and you'll succeed.

More importantly, getting rid of the pull-ups is sending a clear message to your child that you really expect them to succeed. Remember, we transmit messages through our body language and our actions as well as our words.

BEDTIME CHECKLIST

- Repeat clenching muscles and balloon exercises as often as you like. ☐

- Visualise gate on bladder and close it tight. ☐

- Set volume control on HIGH. ☐

- Speak 'auto-pilot phrases' out loud. ☐

- Programme Sat Nav ☐

- Listen to audio recording. ☐

RECORDING SUCCESS

Keeping track of progress will spur your child on to even greater success. Tell your child that from now on he is going to have to behave a little like a 'detective' – noticing small changes, collecting evidence and proof that he is moving closer and closer each day to his goal.

It's going to be important to keep a record of all successes, big and small, rather than simply keeping a record of dry nights or wet nights. There may be the occasional wet night and, if this does happen, your child's 'detective' powers will need to be even more special.

Record any proof or evidence of successfully keeping to the system and leaving old habits and behaviours behind. This could be as simple as listening to the recording before bedtime and carrying out some of the visualisation exercises. Even the act of going to bed without wearing protective pants is a huge step forward and deserves to be recorded as success. So, even if an accident occurs, there is still 'progress' that can be captured.

Some children report that, on occasions, although they didn't quite make it to the bathroom in time, they did wake up in time to be aware of wetting the bed. If in the past, your child would normally have slept right the way through, then they have made 'progress'. It demonstrates that the messages are getting through, the system is working and they'll most probably be dry the next night.

Let's not forget, each small step forward, however small, is one step further forward in the process of having dry nights forever. The more 'success steps' you can record, the more you'll be helping your child to reach their overall goal.

You can either record your child's progress in the spaces provided below or you can buy a separate notebook or diary for your child to use. As well as making a note of events on a daily basis, your child can also use this book to remind themselves of how different life will be in the future.

Encourage your child to be creative – maybe drawing more pictures or sticking in photos of friends he'd like to have sleepovers with, or even pictures of places he may go to on overnight school trips.

Remember, all the children who have used this system with me have been really successful, really quickly.

MY SUCCESS RECORD

These were my successes today:

Date : . . . .

. . . .

. . . .

Date : . . . .

. . . .

. . . .

Date : . . . .

. . ..

. . . .

Date : . . . .

.. . .

.. . .

<u>MY SUCCESS RECORD</u>

These were my successes today:

Date : . . . .

. . . .

. . . .

Date : . . . .

. . . .

. . . .

Date : . . . .

. . . .

. . . .

Date : . . . .

. . . .

. . . .

MY SUCCESS RECORD

These were my successes today:

Date : . . . .

. . . .

. . . .

Date : . . . .

. . . .

. . . .

Date : . . . .

. . . .

. . . .

Date : . . . .

. . . .

. . . .

COOLING OFF PERIOD

Once your child has been dry every night for two weeks, you can begin winding the activities down. I suggest that the hypnotic recording is listened to just once or twice a week.

You can also review some of the exercises a couple of times during the week. It's very likely that your child will have got into a routine and will automatically repeat most of the exervises, without needing a reminder.

If your child continues to be dry, you'll be able to reduce to just once a week and see how things go.

CELEBRATING SUCCESS

Having successfully worked your way through this programme, you and your child will be able to look forward to that new future with 'dry beds forever'.

This is not magic, but you might be surprised to discover that it might *seem* like magic ....

Enjoy those sleepovers!

Alicia

FREQUENTLY ASKED QUESTIONS

Here are some of the most common questions I get asked by parents who ask me to help their children with their bedwetting problems. This list isn't exhaustive and if there is something specific to your child, please feel free to contact me through my website – www.aliciaeaton.co.uk   . I can't always guarantee a personal reply but I will be updating my Bedwetting EXTRA section on the website regularly.

Q. At what age do children usually become dry at night?

A. There's a complex co-ordination that needs to develop between nerves and muscles in order to control the bladder. This has usually taken place by the age of 5 but some children take a little longer. If your child has reached his or her 6th birthday and still regularly wets the bed, it's a good idea to consider this system to help them become dry.

Q. How old does my child have to be to use this system?

A. Your child will need to be old enough to understand the problem and how they have a part to play in treating themselves and this will vary from child to child. All the techniques described in this book are suitable for use with young children and I have worked in similar ways with children as young as four years.

Q. What happens if we miss doing the activities on one of the days?

A. Continue to work through the system on the next available day. Ensure your child can remember the previous activities well enough before moving on to the next one. Don't attempt to 'catch up' by doing two day's activities in one and remember to alter any dates you may have marked in the calendar. However, once your child starts to listen to the CD, it's best not to miss a day for at least one week.

Q. I can't eliminate all pull-up pants from the house as my child's 3 year old sister is still wearing them at night. Is this a problem?

A. It's worth finding a new place to store younger siblings' protective night pants, perhaps even providing a new box or container for them to clearly indicate who they belong to. If they share a bedroom do store them as far away as possible.

Q. My child has been dry for 6 nights but wet on the 7th. It was the same story the following week – dry for 6 nights but wet again on the 7th. Should I be thinking about doing something differently?

A. No – your child has had 12 dry nights out of 14. That's fantastic progress – you've clearly being doing everything right and there's no need to think about changing anything. Remember to focus on your child's successes rather than any accidents that may occur along the way.

Q. I can't seem to get my child to follow one of the visualisation exercises – is this going to be a problem?

A. The more exercises your child can take part in, the better – however, it's not essential to follow each one in order to have this process work. It's important for your child to have an understanding of how the mind and body work closely together and it's also important for your child to listen to the CD for several days. Thereafter, there is a degree of flexibility in the system. Whilst I believe it's best to work through all the activities, I have had children who have become completely dry by just listening to my CD and doing no more.

RESOURCES – NAMES AND ADDRESSES

Alicia Eaton – appointments, books and CDs –
www.aliciaeaton.co.uk
www.stopbedwettingin7days.co.uk

The General Hypnotherapy Standards Council –
register of qualified hypnotherapists:
www.general-hypnotherapy-register.com

ERIC – Education and Resources for Improving
Childhood Continence - www.eric.org.uk

Paul McKenna - books and resources
www.paulmckenna.com

Michael Neill - success coaching and more
www.geniuscatalyst.com

The Society of NLP - www.purenlp.com

The Montessori Society – www.montessori-uk.org

NOTES

Also from MX Publishing

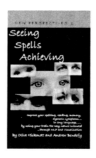

Seeing Spells Achieving

The UK's leading NLP book for learning difficulties including dyslexia.

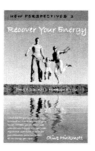

Recover Your Energy

NLP for Chronic Fatigue, ME and tiredness.

More NLP books at www.mxpublishing.co.uk

Lightning Source UK Ltd.
Milton Keynes UK
UKOW03f033120112

185242UK00001B/21/P